I0420153

HOME REMEDIES

Natural Home Remedies Everyone Should Know For The Most Common Health Conditions

Fhilcar Faunillan

Copyright by Content Arcade Publishing
All rights reserved.

This book aims to provide exact and reliable information about the topic covered. The information herein is for informational purposes solely and is universal as so. The presentation of the data comes with no contract or any guarantee assurance. The publisher is not required to render accounting, officially permitted, or otherwise qualified services. If advice is necessary, legal or professional, an expert individual in the profession should be ordered.

From a Declaration of Principles which was accepted and approved equally by a Committee of the American Bar Association and a Committee of Publishers and Associations.

In no way it is legal to duplicate, reproduce, or transmit any part of this book in either printed or electronic format. Recording and storage of this publication are strictly prohibited unless with written permission from the publisher. All rights reserved.

The trademarks used in this book is without permission or backing by the trademark owner. All trademarks and brands contained in this book are for clarifying purposes only and are owned by the owners themselves, not connected with this publication.

Table of Contents

Introduction

To most people, health and overall well-being are the primary concern. Even though how health-conscious we get, there will be times when we have to deal with common health problems like cuts, bruises, acne, and annoying warts, to name a few. And while some of these can be easily brushed aside, some can be bothersome and more prone to infection. That is why learning how to make your own natural home remedies is extremely helpful. Besides having such treatments within your reach, you can also save money because you do not need to go to the doctor for these minor health concerns.

In these modern times, people have become so dependent on pharmaceutical products. While these can give you immediate relief, the complications that come with taking these chemical-based medicines are not something that you can easily ignore. You have probably heard of some pharmaceutical lawsuits; instead of providing relief, some medications have worsened the patient's conditions.

Even though these natural home remedies are generally safe, people who have health problems that are more serious or severe are highly recommended to see their doctor immediately to get the proper advice and treatment they need.

As you go through the pages of this book, you will be amazed that most of the ingredients needed for preparing these home remedies are readily available in your home. You can find them in your kitchen or garden, and since they are natural, they are proven to be without any side effects.

I hope you'll enjoy reading this book!

Chapter 1

Common Foot Conditions, Remedies, and Care

Often, we give the least priority to our feet. We focus mainly on our face and other body parts. But mind you, our feet are among the most overworked body parts – they carry our weight and are also prone to injuries. Here are some of the most common foot conditions and their corresponding remedies.

#1 Cracked Heels

You have been familiar with cracked heels; this usually occurs in summer due to too much dryness on the feet. Also known as fissures, cracking of heels is embarrassing and painful, especially if the cut runs deeper into the skin. If you love wearing open footwear, then you would likely be embarrassed as people would notice this unlikely sight of your feet. Not only is his common among adults, but this can affect youngsters too. Adults, however, are likely to experience this because of aging and overexposure to dryness. Aside from these factors, having a poor and unhealthy lifestyle can contribute to having cracked heels too. Add to that list hypothyroidism, poor foot hygiene, as well as diabetes. The list of the contributing factors can be lengthy.

Remedies

1. *Milk and Honey Moisturizer + Exfoliator*

    Milk works best for the skin. Adding honey to it can make milk a complete exfoliant and moisturizer in one. Because honey contains antibacterial and anti-fungal properties, it is best in treating athlete's foot and other related conditions. Prepare a basin and mix well 2 cups of milk and a cup of honey, then soak your feet for about 15 minutes. You can also warm the liquid if desired for a more comfortable feeling but make sure that you do not heat it much because it will burn and dry your feet. Wash your feet afterward and pat it dry. Repeat this twice a week.

2. *Glycerin and Rosewater Moisturizer*

Glycerin is widely used, especially in cosmetic products, and is an effective moisturizer. Combining it with rosewater makes it a perfect cracked heels solution. The latter ingredient contains antioxidant and anti-inflammatory properties and is also known to be a good antiseptic. Not to mention, it is rich in A, B3, C, D, and E vitamins. You can mix a teaspoon of glycerin to a teaspoon of rosewater and massage it gently on your feet, focusing on the affected areas. Apply it on your feet and wrap it all night, wearing clean cotton socks to lock in moisture.

The solution can also be utilized to soak your feet. Soak your feet in a mixture of glycerin, rosewater, a teaspoon salt, lemon juice, and half a basin of warm water, then wipe it dry.

3. *Rice Flour Exfoliating Scrub*

One way to remove dry and dead skin on your feet and smooth it out is by exfoliating it using your very own rice flour exfoliating scrub. To make the scrub, mix well two teaspoons of apple cider vinegar, two teaspoons of honey, three tablespoons of rice flour, and a few drops of olive oil in a small basin or bowl. Before applying, make sure you have soaked your feet in a pool of warm water for about 20 minutes to soften your skin. Gently rub the scrub on your feet, focusing on the target areas. Repeat this at least twice a week for better results.

4. *Virgin Coconut Oil (VCO) and other Oils (Almond, Olive, Grapeseed, and Sesame) for Massage*

Massaging your heels and feet not only soothes your walkers but helps in regulating the circulation of the blood, especially when essentials oils are used. These natural moisturizers help in healing cracked heels. You can use VCO alone or mix all these oils and massage unto your feet, concentrating on the most affected areas for about 10 minutes, then locking in moisture by wearing clean cotton socks.

5. *ABC (Avocado-Banana-Coconut) Paste*

Avocado is known worldwide to contain natural fatty acids. In many diets, it is incorporated into meals as it has essential oils as well as fat-soluble vitamins. The avocado oil can help repair worn-out tissues and give your skin the natural glow. To prepare the mask, mash together one banana, half an avocado, and coconut meat (about the same quantity as the banana), then apply the paste directly on your feet, carefully massaging it. Allow it to stay for 20 minutes before washing it off with lukewarm water and wiping it dry.

6.   *Epsom Salt Soak*

Epsom Salt Soak is known for being a natural cure for various skin problems. Epsom salt is can easily be absorbed by the skin, soothe your tired feet, relieve the athlete's foot, and cure fungal infections. A 10-minute foot soak therapy consisting of warm water and half a cup of Epsom salt can heal your cracked heels. If you have pumice, rub your feet using it, then dry it well. Afterward, rub the whole area with petroleum jelly and tuck it in all night to retain moisture by wearing clean, cottony socks. Repeat this twice a week.

7.   *Vinegar Soak*

Vinegar, especially apple cider, is useful in treating various skin conditions. Direct application on the skin can, however, result in dryness. For that reason, I do not recommend that you use it directly on your skin. Soak and gently rub your feet with a pumice stone for about 15 minutes in a mixture of a quarter cup of vinegar, about the same amount of olive oil, and half a basin of warm water. Dry it with a clean towel and moisturize.

8. *Paraffin Wax*

Apart from the countless benefits, it provides a cure for cracked feet and removal of dead skin; paraffin wax is also used to soothe tiredness on the joints and muscles. Add mustard oil or VCO to melted paraffin wax. Once cooled, coat it on your feet all night and tuck it in by wearing cottony socks. Do this daily for up to 15 days to achieve the best results.

9. *Papaya-Lemon Mask*

Lemon is known for its exfoliating properties and its effectiveness in getting off dead skin. Papaya, on the other hand, has enzymes that can smoothen the surface. When combined to form a paste, it can be an effective remedy for cracked heels. To prepare, mix mashed papaya and lemon juice and apply the mixture directly on your feet. Allow it to stand for 15 minutes before washing your walkers with warm water mixed with lemon juice. Soak for another 15 minutes. You may use a pumice stone to scrub off dead skin and pat it dry with a clean towel.

10. *Jojoba and Oatmeal Mask*

With both having moisturizing properties, jojoba oil, and oatmeal can you're your skin amazing benefits. Mix a teaspoon of oatmeal and the desired amount of oil to form a thick paste and apply it directly on your feet leaving it for 20 minutes. Rinse it off with warm water and pat it dry with a clean towel.

11. *DIY Foot Ointment*

Applying ointment on your feet overnight can give you a soothing feeling and help in moisturizing your parched walkers. Wear cottony socks to tuck in moisture. To create your own ointment, you can mix a quarter cup of coconut oil and the same amount of magnesium flakes as well as Shea butter, two tablespoons of boiling water, and three tablespoons of beeswax.

#2 Athlete's Foot

An infection caused by the fungus, Tinea pedis, athlete's foot is characterized by having inflamed, itchy, burning, and stingy feet, especially in the groin area. Scaly and white patches are highly noticeable. The presence of the fungus can also cause redness.

While this condition is present in the foot area, it can also affect your fingers. That is why avoid contact as much as possible; and do not forget to wash your hands thoroughly.

Keep your feet dry, avoid footwear that uses synthetic materials, wear cotton socks, and do not wear your shoes the day after you have worn them. Allow them to dry completely as wet and dark areas are a great host for fungus.

Remedies

1. *Organic Ginger Rinse*

    Aside from having strong anti-fungal properties, ginger can also give your walkers a spicy yet pleasant smell. Add about an ounce of freshly chopped ginger to a cup of boiling water. Simmer it for 15 minutes. Allow it to cool and apply it directly to your feet. Make sure you have cleaned your feet well before using ginger. For best results, the application should be twice a day.

2. *Organic Tea Tree Oil Soak*

Tea tree oil can soothe your feet. It can also destroy fungus, especially in profoundly affected areas, and stop it from spreading. Add 40 drops to your foot bath. Soak your feet for 10-15 minutes and pat it try.

3. *Raw Virgin Coconut/Sesame Oil Swab*

These oils contain anti-fungal properties. Wet a cotton ball and apply the oil on your feet directly, especially in the most affected areas. Do this twice a day.

4. *Lemon Rinse*

Lemon has deodorizing properties and can lessen foot odor caused by athlete's foot. Soak your feet for 15 minutes in a basin half-filled with lukewarm water mixed with half a cup of lemon juice. Pat your feet dry after with a clean towel. Do this twice daily to achieve better results.

5. *Baking Soda Paste*

An anti-fungal and bacteria killer at the same time, baking soda is very useful in treating athlete's foot. To prepare the paste, add 1-part water to 3 parts baking soda. Stir until a thick paste is formed and rub it gently on your feet. Do not forget to include the area between your toes. Allow the paste to dry and run water on your feet, then pat it dry. You can also sprinkle your shoes with baking soda before wearing them.

6. *Garlic and Olive Oil Rub*

You may think that your feet would become stinky by applying garlic on it, but that is a very effective deodorizer. Add olive oil to crushed garlic and use it directly on your feet. Allow it to stay all night by wearing cottony socks.

7. *Himalayan Crystal Salt and Apple Cider Solution*

This solution is very useful in treating athlete's foot as acid does not allow fungi to thrive. In half a basin of lukewarm water, add half a cup of organic apple cider vinegar to 2 tablespoons of Himalayan crystal salt. Soak your feet for 15 minutes. You can also use this as a foot spray after a shower but do not forget to wipe your feet dry applying. If you decide to spray it on your footwear as well, be sure to dry them thoroughly before using it.

8. *Cornstarch Rub*

Browned cornstarch absorbs all moisture. Thus, applying this to your feet will keep it dry. Lightly brown half a cup of cornstarch on a pre-heated oven (325 degrees). Be careful not to burn it. Rub it on your feet, leave for 10 minutes, and then wipe it off with a clean, dry towel.

9. *Oregano Tea Soak*

You can make oregano tea by boiling 4 ounces of leaves in half a basin of water. Soak your feet in oregano tea thrice daily up to three weeks.

10. *Plain Yogurt*

Buy yogurt that has live acidophilus as that is effective in fighting against fungi and bacteria. Rub it on your feet using a cotton swab and allow it to dry. Rinse it off with lukewarm water and pat your feet with a clean, dry towel. Eat yogurt as well for a faster recovery.

#3 Sweaty Feet

Hyperhidrosis or excessive sweating can be very embarrassing, but there are several ways to treat this. Sweaty feet can be a home for fungi that can cause a foul odor. Cleaning your feet and scrubbing it regularly will help you avoid having smelly feet. Wearing clean cottony socks and daily changing of socks and shoes are likewise recommended.

Remedies

1. *Tomato Juice Scrub*

   Soak your feet daily for about half an hour in a mixture of lukewarm water and 3 cups of tomato juice.

2. *Baking Soda Soak*

   Regular daily soaking of your walkers for 20 minutes in a mixture of lukewarm water and 2 cups of baking soda can give you instant relief.

3. *Apple Cider Bath*

> Soak your feet in half a basin of water with half a cup of apple cider vinegar for 15 minutes to reduce perspiration. Wash your feet after using only mild soap and dry it off.

#4 Ingrown Toenails

Commonly known as an ingrown toenail, onychocryptosis is a painful nail disease that is accompanied by swelling and redness of the area around it. You can notice that your nail grows on either or both sides of the nail bed, and in worst cases, you may see a growth of tissue or a yellowish fluid on the affected area. Wearing tight shoes, trimming your nails very short, improper trimming (not straight across), and toe injury, among others, are the common causes of ingrown toenails. In worst cases, an operation may be necessary.

Remedies

1. *Apple Cider*

> Apple cider is a powerful cure to many conditions. You can apply it directly to your

ingrown toenail or use it as a foot soak. Add half a cup to half a basin of water. You can also consume a tablespoon daily. If you find its taste intolerable, mix it with honey to cure the taste.

2. *Oregano Essential Oil*

Oregano essential oil can give you immediate relief from pain. Mix it with olive oil and apply it directly to the affected area. However, if you are pregnant or having some allergies, you need to refrain from using this remedy.

3. *Lemon*

Lemon is likewise a cure to various health problems. To use this remedy, place a thin lemon slice on your toenail and bandage it. Leave it overnight.

4. *Epsom Salt*

Epsom salt helps in softening the skin on the affected area so you can quickly draw the toenail from being buried on the surface. Soak your feet twice daily for 20 minutes in a basin of lukewarm water with Epsom salt.

5. *Lavender/Tea Tree Essential Oil*

Directly apply these essential oils on your ingrown toenail as these serve as natural antibiotics.

#5 Corns and Calluses

Corns and calluses occur as a result of protecting your feet from rubbing against surfaces, even your toes or shoes.

Corns can be either be soft or hard. Hard corns are cone-shaped and point into the skin, while soft ones are between toes. Corns occur as a result of pressure being exerted by the bones of one toe against the other. The hard ones can be found on the outer sides or top of the toes as a result of friction as your toe rubs against your shoes.

On the other hand, calluses are found on flat surfaces of the foot, which often rubs against your shoes as

when you wear high heels.

Remedies

1. *Apple Cider Soak*

   For calluses, soak your feet for 15 minutes in half a basin with lukewarm soapy water and a cup of apple cider, then rub it off with a pumice stone.

2. *Castor Oil*

   Dab castor oil on corns after soaking your feet in apple cider. You can use a cotton swab and leave it bandaged. Wear cotton socks to lock moisture and repeat this procedure for ten days until corns have peeled off.

3. *Bread and Apple Cider Pad*

   Using stale bread and apple cider can be very useful in treating corns and calluses. Soak the bread in apple cider, then place it on the affected area. You can use adhesive tape to lock it in overnight and wear cotton socks. You'll be surprised to see your corn or callus gone the moment you wake up.

4. *Onion*

   Soak a slice of onion in white vinegar in a glass container for at least 12 hours. Leave it during the day in a warm place. In the evening, use the onion to cover the affected area. Leave it covered overnight by securing it with a bandage. Repeat this process until it softens.

5. *Lemon Peel*

Lemon peels are also useful in removing corns and calluses. Have a slice about the size of your target (toe) and place it on the area. Utilizing a bandage and wearing cotton socks overnight will help in keeping it in place. Please continue with the process until it disappears.

#6 Plantar Warts

Plantar warts are rough skin growths caused by human papillomavirus (HPV). They appear on your feet's soles. While most warts do not seem to bother you at all, they are just embarrassing and contagious.

Remedies

1. *Lemon Squeeze*

   Lemon can be very useful in removing plantar warts. Squeeze it directly on the affected area and allow it to dry. Leave it overnight and repeat the same step for three weeks or until warts are completely gone.

2. *Garlic Rub*

   Crush garlic and rub it directly on the affected area. Allow the garlic to stay overnight and apply the same procedure until the warts are completely gone.

3. *Ginger Press*

   Ginger has been known to remove warts the quickest way, although this is quite tricky. Get cardboard and cut out a hole tracing the wart/infected area. Cut the insides to cover the non-infected regions. Heat some ginger over stove fire and cut it out to reveal the meat. What we need here is the juice. Then press the ginger on the wart while it is still hot and squeeze the ginger. Allow it to dry. Repeat this for the second or third time until you notice that the blemishes are peeling off like thread.

#7 Toenail Fungal Infection

Another common toenail issue is the fungal infection known as onychomycosis. This condition appears first as either a yellow or white spot. You would notice that your toenails easily crumble, become distorted, dull, thickened, and darker as the infection digs deeper. This process emits an unpleasant odor. Unless the fungus spreads, you feel no pain yet. If you notice your toenails to be having this kind of infection, address the issue at once as it can cause further splitting of your toenails, and the worst thing is, you may lose your toenail completely. Poor hygiene, sweaty feet, and exposure to moist environments give the fungus a chance to thrive.

Remedies

1. *Orange/Tea Tree Oil Rub*

   With anti-bacterial and fungicidal properties, orange and tea tree oils are a sure way to treat toenail fungal infection. To prepare the rub, dilute a teaspoon of tea tree oil, then add in half a teaspoon of olive oil and half a teaspoon of orange oil. Dip a cotton ball into the mixture and apply it to the infected area. Always wash your hands afterward. Repeat this twice daily.

2. *Orange/Tea Tree Oil Soak*

When used as a soak, add the mixture to half a basin of lukewarm water and soak your feet for 20 minutes. Dry it off using a clean towel and repeat this procedure twice daily.

3. *Snakeroot Extract*

Snakeroot extract also has anti-fungal properties. Apply this thrice a week in your first month, then twice a week on the second and once a week on the third.

4. *Baking Soda and Vinegar Soak*

An acidic environment does not allow the fungus to thrive. When combined with baking soda, which is also very useful in preventing fungi from spreading and growing, it becomes a very potent solution. To prepare, add five teaspoons of baking soda and a cup of white vinegar to half a basin of water and soak your feet for 15 minutes. Dry them with a clean towel and repeat this twice daily.

Chapter 2

Dreaded Facial and Head Problems

Among our body parts, our face is the most visible. Should you wish to hide any imperfection, covering your face is not easy at all. The face also is the reflection of our outer beauty. It shows one's youthfulness, sophistication and manifests our emotions. As much as we want to have a flawless look, times may come when you come across various facial problems that arise along with age (puberty). That is why we need to consume healthy foods, hydrate well, and practice basic hygiene.

Compiled in this chapter are common facial problems and their respective remedies.

#1 Acne

Termed as Acne Vulgaris, this can be found not only on the face but also in other body parts – chest, shoulders, back, or neck. It can start as our skin's sebaceous/oil glands produce oily secretions. Once the clogging starts, it can result in either blackheads (for bigger pores) or whiteheads (for smaller pores). If it becomes irritated and is inflamed, then pimples develop.

In mild cases, acne is manifested by occasional pimples. If the case is acute, you may notice inflamed papules. In severe cases, cyst-like nodules are present. Acne is a common occurrence to those who reach the age of puberty until their 30's although studies have shown that there are still those who get acne even in their 50's.

Remedies

1. *Green Tea Miracle Detox*

   Present in green tea is Epigallocatechin Gallate (EGCG), an antioxidant that reduces bacterial growth, inflammation, and sebum production, which are the main culprits for acne breakouts. Creating a miracle detox is easy. Steep for five minutes about two teaspoons of loose organic green tea leaves in half a cup of boiling water. Strain the leaves, leaving the water to cool. Using a cotton bud, apply it directly to your face. You may also use green tea bags. Soak it for three minutes, then remove the bag and apply it directly on your face.

2. *Minty Rub*

Mint has menthol, which is both useful as a pain killer and an anti-inflammatory agent. Although this is not the secret formula to cure acne, this minimizes redness and relieves inflammation. All you have to do is crush some fresh mint leaves and rub it directly on your face; then, leave it there for 10 minutes. Rinse it off with cold water, and you will surely feel refreshed.

3. *Honey and Avocado Mask*

Avocados have numerous health benefits. It can quickly provide a cure to dry and flaky skin as it contains antioxidants, healthy fat, moisture, natural oils, and phytochemicals. Basing on that premise, various avocado-based topical solutions have been created, including this honey and avocado mask. Apply directly on your face mashed quarter of an avocado that's mixed with a tablespoon of honey. Leave it on your face for 20 minutes before washing it off with lukewarm water and drying it. I also recommend this to those who have sensitive skin.

4. *Honey and Oatmeal Scrub*

Dead skin cells and excess oils that cause acne may be removed with the use of oatmeal. It can also reduce inflammation. To prepare, add two tablespoons of raw honey to a serving of cooked oats. Once cooled, apply it directly to the face, leaving it for 20 minutes before rinsing your face with lukewarm water and drying it.

5. *Egg White and Avocado Mask*

Excessive skin oil that can clog your pores and cause blackheads and acne can easily be removed with the help of egg white. Avocado, having natural fats, can nourish your skin and is an excellent remedy for dry skin. If you wonder why we came up with such a combination, knowing that their purposes seem contrasting, well, I tell you, this makes the mask great for both dry and oily skin.

To prepare, mash a quarter serving of avocado and one egg white and massage it gently on your face. Make sure to cover all areas, leaving it for 15 minutes before rinsing it off with lukewarm water and drying it.

6. *Cinnamon-Honey-Nutmeg Mask*

This mask is also very easy to prepare. Form a paste by combining honey, freshly grated nutmeg, and cinnamon. Leave the mixture for at least an hour before using it, then let it stay on your face for 15 minutes before rinsing it off with lukewarm water and drying it.

7. *Baking Soda Exfoliant*

An economical way of gently exfoliating your skin is with the use of sodium bicarbonate or baking soda. Exfoliating helps remove dead skin cells and unclogs your pores. Dissolve a teaspoon of baking soda in about the same amount of water, just enough to create a paste. You can also add lemon to it. Place it directly on your acne and leave it there for 5 minutes before rinsing it off with lukewarm water and drying it.

#2 Facial Warts

Warts, which are caused by HPV, can grow anywhere in the body, including the facial area. Flat warts are more common among children and teenagers than in adults. They can develop in the legs and arms, especially in women, and are likewise contagious. They appear to be flatter (as the name suggests) than other warts that appear on the other parts of the body, smaller, smoother, and can be yellowish, brownish, or pinkish.

Remedies

1. *Apple Cider Astringent*

   The mother of all solutions, apple cider, is very effective in giving warts an unpleasant environment. Use a cotton ball when applying it on warts. Allow it to dry. You can have this on a cotton swab for better results and place it on warts, enough to cover the affected area and secure with a bandage. Let it stay all night and wash your face the moment you wake up. Do this daily, and you will notice warts peeling off in a week or so.

Make a careful observation while using this treatment because you might notice some swelling and soreness on your skin. However, that should be normal. If the side effects are no longer tolerable, be sure to stop using this treatment and consult a doctor then.

2. *Vitamin C Crystals Plus Lemon Spot Treatment*

Vitamin C and lemon are both acidic, which can give warts a non-livable environment, thus killing and destroying HPV. To prepare, have enough lemon juice (a few drops) and mix it well with vitamin C crystals. Apply it directly on your wart and secure it with a bandage. Repeat this until warts have entirely peeled off.

3. *Garlic Mask*

Garlic contains allicin, which is a useful antiviral substance and can help you get rid of a wide range of viruses, including HPV. To apply, crush a clove of garlic and use it directly on warts. As much as possible, refrain from having the garlic touch your skin as you may feel soreness and pain. Bandage it and leave it there all night. Repeat this procedure daily until warts would peel off.

4. *Banana Mask*

Banana is rich in an enzyme called proteolytic, which can break down protein, thereby eating up and dissolving facial warts. For this, you will need a banana peel (not the flesh). Scrape the insides of the skin and apply it directly to blemishes. You can hold this for a couple of hours before you rinse your face.

#3 Wrinkles, Dark Circles, and Age Spots

As you age, you will notice wrinkles, dark circles, and age spots around your eyes and facial area. These are the most dreaded signs of aging as they are visible. To prevent having these, get enough sleep, eat healthily, exercise, and brush aside all your worries. A lot of people may have gone through cosmetic surgeries to eliminate them, but just like any condition, you can avoid or get rid of them the natural way.

Remedies

1. *Cucumber Mask*

    Applying refrigerated cucumber slices on your eyes would not only give your peepers a cooling effect but also moisturize it. Wrinkles and dark circles are caused by skin breakage due to dryness. So, provide adequate moisture and give your eyes a refreshing relief.

2. *Avocado Mask*

    Putting mashed avocado under your peepers for 20 minutes can remove wrinkles and dark spots. Avocado is rich in fat and vitamin E, which is needed to nourish your dry skin and prevent the skin from sagging. Do this twice a week, and you'll surely have wrinkle-free skin that glows.

3. *Banana and Yogurt Mask*

    Yogurt and banana are not just good when taken in by the body but can also be an active facial mask. It contains vitamin A, which effectively removes blemishes and dark spots, vitamin B to give you a youthful glow and cures wrinkles, vitamin E to protect your skin from the harmful UV rays and effectively fights free radicals, as well as potassium which is vital for cell hydration. To prepare, mix these ingredients – one whole mashed banana, a teaspoon of yogurt, and a teaspoon of orange juice – and apply it directly on your face, leaving it for 20 minutes.

4. *Coconut/Olive Oil Miracle*

Coconut is known as the 'tree of life.' True to such fact, this tree has countless uses and benefits, especially when it comes to health. Coconut oil contains antioxidants that combat the formation of free radicals. Free radicals, as we know, cause deterioration among things in the surroundings, which include, among others, the human body. One effect is aging. As it prevents the formation of free radicals, you are therefore free from experiencing wrinkles and other age-associated conditions. Olive oil, on the other hand, contains vitamins A and E.

A daily dose of these vitamins is needed by your skin to achieve that youthful glow you so desire for years. Apply a tablespoon at least once a day by gently massaging it directly on your face and wear it on your face overnight for better results. Olive oil can also be used in the morning as it contains UV protecting properties. Never set out in the sun without having a strong shield against its powerful rays.

5. *Lemon-Egg White-Honey Mask*

Egg whites are very useful for maintaining your skin's tightness, thus preventing sagging. During the process of tightening, your pores are shrunk, thereby reducing excessive pore oil secretion. Therefore, protein-rich egg whites are ideal for aging skin, too, as it hastens tissue growth and repair. They contain lysozyme, which destroys acne-causing bacteria. Aside from that, potassium, which helps moisturize the skin cells, is also present in enough amounts along with magnesium that helps keep your skin radiant looking and delays the aging process, and vitamin B2, which fights free radicals and toxins that cause wrinkles. To prepare, mix a teaspoon of freshly squeezed lemon with half a spoon of honey and one egg white. Please do not leave it overnight. As your skin tightens, rinse it off to avoid sagging and protect your eyes from having eye bags. Imagine having your skin stretched so much. That's why extra care is necessary when using this remedy.

6. *Water Hydration*

Water is the world's best solvent. It is also the secret to attaining the fountain of youth. Drink at least eight glasses of water daily to hydrate your skin and face. While you hydrate outside, never miss the insides too. Aside from that, regular water intake helps in flushing the toxins out of your body.

7. *Tomato*

Instantly brighten your skin and give it a youthful glow by applying tomato not just on your face but neck too. Daily consumption can also make your cheeks turn naturally red. Not only that, it can effectively eliminate wrinkles and tighten your skin.

8. *Ginger and Honey Rub*

Ginger, when combined with honey, becomes an effective rub for increasing blood circulation around the area. It is also a moisturizer and humectant in one. To prepare, mix thoroughly half a teaspoon of honey and a teaspoon of ginger extract. Apply it directly to your wrinkles and dark circles. Gently massage the area affected for about 10 minutes and rinse your face with water after that. Do this daily.

9. *Pineapple Juice Exfoliant and Astringent*

Alpha hydroxyl acid (AHA), which is essential for skin rejuvenation and wrinkle treatment, can be found in pineapple juice. Bromelain, an active enzyme, is a natural form of AHA. Pineapple juice can also be an effective treatment for inflammation. Apply pineapple juice directly on the affected area, leaving it there for 20 minutes before rinsing it off. Do this daily to achieve the best results. Not only will you be able to eliminate those undesirable signs of aging but prevent its early onset.

10. *Rosemary Essential Oil*

Essential oils have a lot of health benefits, including skin nourishment and protection. The other is wrinkle prevention. Apply this under your eyes and massage gently to eliminate wrinkles and prevent the formation of aging lines. Make this a daily habit.

11. *Rice Powder Mask*

This mask will not only remove wrinkles, tighten your skin, and correct the visible signs of aging but will also make your skin naturally glowing. Mix the rice powder, milk, and rose water to form a thick paste and apply it directly to your face. Leave it there for 20 minutes, then rinse off with cold water.

12. *Topical Vitamin C*

Overexposure to sunlight can significantly damage your skin. You would notice fine lines and discoloration with occasional flaking or dryness. Nourish your skin not just by consuming vitamin C for faster cell repair but applying topical vitamin C to exfoliate.

#4 Puffy Eyes

Looking at yourself in the mirror and seeing those bulging or sagging eye bags can be frustrating. Puffy eyes or what we commonly call eye bags can be normal to some individuals. People with puffy eyes experience swelling of the orbits (tissues around the eyes). Thus, in medical terms, it is called periorbital puffiness. Puffiness can be attributed to various factors, including crying, allergies, oversleeping or lack of sleep, over fatigue, diet, and a lot more. While some causes can only result in temporary puffiness, others, including skin disorders, improper functioning tear glands, and some diseases, can pose an alarm to you. Surgery is required in severe cases of puffiness.

Remedies

1. *Cucumber Eye Mask*

   You surely are familiar with cucumber eye masks. Cucumbers contain enzymes and powerful astringent properties that effectively relieve stressed skin, tighten it, and is also an excellent anti-inflammatory. Thus, it can be an excellent treatment for eye bags, including wrinkles and dark circles. All you need to do is chill a piece of cucumber for 10 minutes and cut into thick slices. Cover each of your eyes with one slice and then leave it there for about 15 minutes or until the coldness is gone. This mask will give you much time to relax, too, as you close your peepers for a little while. Do this daily.

2. *Egg Whites Plus Witch Hazel*

To iterate, egg whites can easily tighten your skin and eliminate even the slightest wrinkles. Witch hazel is likewise useful in skin tightening. These skin tightening properties are essential for removing puffiness too. Beat egg whites and a few drops of witch hazel together until stiff and apply it directly under your eyes. Wait for it to dry for about 15 minutes, then wash it off with cold water. Repeat this procedure until the puffiness disappears.

3. *Hydrate with Nothing Else but Water*

Water is perhaps the easiest and the cost-friendly remedy. To iterate, drinking at least eight glasses of water daily not only gives your cells a boost but adds a glow to your skin. Water flushes toxins out of the body and eliminates puffiness as there are rare chances of water retention, which can lead to swelling of the body parts, including the under-eye area. For best results, avoid salty foods as much as possible as salt causes the body to retain much water—Shun from drinking soda and other carbonated drinks, including caffeine. It would also be best if you avoided alcohol as they give you the opposite effect, which is dehydration.

4. *Potato Starch Patch*

Another means to remove eye bags is with the use of potatoes. Potatoes contain starch, which has anti-inflammatory properties that effectively relieves swelling in the under-eye area. It's so easy to prepare. Peel the skin of a medium-sized potato, then wash and dry it properly. Cut the potato into thin slices, then wrap it in a clean cotton cloth. Use it as an eye mask and leave it for about 20 minutes. Do this daily until you notice that the puffiness is gone. It is useful in treating dark circles too.

5. *Tea Bag Masks*

Green tea has many health benefits. So, whenever you drink a cup of tea, don't throw those tea bags away. Refrigerate two used teabags (cooled) and place them on your eyelids for 15 minutes. It will not only relieve your eyes from puffiness and redness, but it can also make your skin glow.

6. *Cold Metal Spoons*

The use of cold spoons is also an easy and economical eye bag remedy. Yes, you read it right. Although you may think twice of using this remedy, it has been proven by many who have tried this; myself included. Take out six metal spoons and refrigerate it for 15 minutes. You can place it in the freezer for faster cooling if you want. Now, take two of that and put it on your eye bags. Leave it on the area until the coldness is gone and replace it with the other two chilled spoons. It may look funny, but the idea behind this is when you put a cold pack on your eye bags, it can help relieve tired eyes and relax the blood vessels. In effect, your skin will tighten up, and you would be able to get rid of the puffiness.

7. *Teething Rings*

Refrigerating teething rings and placing it on your eye bags works in the same way as the metal spoons. Repeat the procedure daily until you have finally relieved yourself from unwanted puffiness.

8. *Avocado Mask*

The avocado works best in skin enhancing. Remove all your blemishes, dark circles, wrinkles, and eye bags by placing cold, ripe avocado slices as an eye mask.

9. Almond and Milk Paste

Milk and ground almonds are great finishers. Not only are these good in removing puffiness, but these also nourish your eyes and skin as well, giving your skin around the eye area a clearer complexion.

#5 Clogged Pores

Your skin has pores. You might barely notice it because they are not very visible, but some people have large pores. If you are one of those people who do not have to worry about having visible pores, then consider yourself lucky in that aspect. Nevertheless, you still need to check out for clogged pores, which is the result of the accumulation of dirt, oil, dead skin, and other undesirable debris. Another cause of clogging of pores is inflammation due to excess white blood cells.

Why is it necessary to unclog your pores? That to prevent acne and blackheads. Not only are these embarrassing, but can cause ugliness on the overall look of your face. Well, who does not want to look flawless and feel beautiful? Everyone does; that is why you need to get rid of these impurities to look younger and have smoother skin.

Remedies

1. *Lemon and Brown Sugar Scrub*

   Lemon and sugar are natural exfoliants. Besides, lemon is an excellent antioxidant to unclog pores effectively. To prepare, mix lemon to about two tablespoons of sugar and a few drops of water, slightly crushing it in the process of blending to make the crystals turn powdery. Gently scrub it in a circular motion on your face, especially around the nasal area, where dirt can mostly accumulate. Do this once per week for better results.

2. *Raw Honey Scrub*

   Honey contains antibacterial properties and can help open pores to unclog it and successfully eliminate accumulated dirt and oil. Gently massage your skin with raw honey and leave it for 10 minutes before rinsing it off with lukewarm water.

3. *Honey and Baking Soda Exfoliant Cream*

Adding two tablespoons of honey to a teaspoon of baking soda can help unclog your pores and exfoliate in the process. I highly recommend this cream to those with blackheads. Massage your skin using this exfoliant cream for about 10 minutes, then rinse it off.

4. *Honey and Cinnamon Cream*

Cinnamon has skin lightening properties. Mix two tablespoons of it to three tablespoons of honey for a complete rejuvenation and lightening cream, gently massage your skin for about 15 minutes and then rinse it off with lukewarm water. Do this once weekly.

5. *Honey and Yogurt Mask*

Prepare two teaspoons of yogurt and an equal amount of honey. Drop a teaspoon of jojoba oil, then mix them thoroughly to form a paste. Gently massage it on your face for about 15 minutes, then rinse it off with water.

6. *Almond, Egg and Lemon Scrub*

Make an instant scrub that would help you in unclogging pores, exfoliating, and enhancing your skin. All you need to do is whip an egg white until smooth, put in the fridge for about 10 minutes, and then add lemon and crushed almonds. Gently massage the scrub on your face in circular motions for 15 minutes, then rinse it off with water.

7. *Steaming Your Face*

By far, this is the most affordable means to effectively unclog pores and remove impurities and unwanted particles. But it would help if you observed extra care so as not to burn your face instead. Boil a pot of water. Once steam starts to come out, remove the bowl from the stove and lean over the pan to have the steam on your face. Make sure to cover your head with a towel so that all the vapor goes to your face. Remain in that position for about 15 minutes to complete open pores. Dry your skin off with a clean cloth afterward and moisturize your skin. Do this twice weekly.

8. *Baking Soda Facial Cleanser*

Known for its countless household use, baking soda is an effective exfoliant and a good skin pH regulator at the same time. Exfoliation unclogs pores during the process and eliminates unwanted particles, dead skin cells, and other impurities. To prepare, add a teaspoon of water to 2 teaspoons of baking soda, mixing well until you form a paste. Massage it gently on your face for 5 minutes, then rinse it off with lukewarm water. As a caveat, don't use this as a daily cleanser, though. Use it only once weekly.

9. *Honey, Baking Soda, Lemon, and Cinnamon Cleanser*

If you wish to add some twist to your regular baking soda cleanser, adding a teaspoon of cinnamon, lemon juice, and five tablespoons of honey to it is highly recommended. Gently massage the mixture on your face and use this regimen twice weekly.

#6 Dandruff

A common scalp condition characterized by having flaky dead skin is dandruff. It is difficult to treat this, and often, it becomes a source of embarrassment as flakes fill your dark clothes around your shoulders as they fall off or fly like dust. In more severe conditions, dandruff can also be visible in some body parts like the eyebrows, ear canal, and forehead. You need to quickly address this issue as dryness can cause your scalp to turn reddish, itchy, and in worst cases, it can lead to permanent hair loss.

One way to avoid having dandruff is rinsing your hair, making sure your scalp gets a thorough cleaning and not just the rest of your body. Another is changing your shampoo every other week.

Remedies

1. *Apple Cider Spray*

   Apple cider is an excellent anti-dandruff treatment. Its acidity changes your scalp's pH, thereby giving yeast, fungi, and bacteria an undesirable environment. You can apply this before going to the shower. To prepare, combine a cup of water with an equal amount of apple cider. Transfer it to a spray bottle and spray it directly on your scalp. Retain the apple cider on your scalp for an hour by wrapping your head with a shower cap, then wash your hair afterward. Repeat this twice weekly.

2. *Tea Tree on Your Shampoo*

Tea tree oil stops the spread of dandruff. To apply, add a few drops to your regular shampoo each time you wash your hair.

3. *Baking Soda Shampoo*

With its anti-fungal properties, baking soda is useful for treating dandruff too. Apply a handful of baking soda on your wet hair and massage it thoroughly on your scalp for 10 minutes. Run cold water on your hair. Do not use shampoo. You may notice dryness on your hair but do not worry as that is just temporary. The dullness will soon be replaced with luster once the flakes are gone.

4. *Yogurt*

Plain yogurt is right for your hair, plus it fights off fungi that cause dandruff. Apply it directly on your scalp after you have wet your hair.

Leave it for 15 minutes before washing your hair with a minimal amount of shampoo.

5. *Coconut Oil*

Nourish your scalp by applying coconut oil to it before washing your hair. Be sure not to use it on your hair – just your scalp and rinse it off once or twice to remove the coconut oil.

6. *C.H.O.Y. Scrub*

For this, you will be making a super powerful scrub. Mix three teaspoons of yogurt to 2 teaspoons of each coconut oil, honey, and olive oil to create a paste. Make sure it is thick enough to hold on to your scalp. Should it appear thin and soft, you can add honey and yogurt to make it thicker. Once you have the paste, apply it directly on your scalp, massaging it gently to penetrate the roots of your hair for 10 minutes. Allow it to sit on your scalp for another 20 minutes. You can also sit under a steamer for better results. Doing so will open the pores on your scalp and help in promoting blood circulation. Rinse your hair, and if you want, you can wash it off with a mild shampoo.

7. *Lemony Egg Yolks*

Egg yolk is not only effective in eliminating dandruff but also in preventing hair fall and giving your hair its natural shine. Mix a whole egg yolk thoroughly to a teaspoon of lemon and massage unto scalp. Leave for an hour before shampooing your hair and lock it with a shower cap. Be sure not to leave it for more than the recommended duration as eggs can easily smell bad.

8. *Aloe Vera Hair Gel*

Aloe Vera is known to give your hair the glow it needs and is very useful in treating dandruff. To prepare, you will need an Aloe Vera leaf, of course. Slice it off halfway (not all the way through). Scoop out the gel. You can also add coconut oil and vitamin E if you like, but the Aloe Vera gel is enough, though. Massage it on your scalp gently for 15 minutes. Consumption of Aloe Vera juice is also encouraged for better results.

#7 Airplane Ear

Aerotitis media, barotitis media, or ear barotrauma are the medical terms used to refer to the condition known as airplane ear. As the name suggests, you experience pressure exerted on your middle ear tissues and eardrum when you ride a plane. This condition happens every time you encounter an imbalance in the air pressure in the environment, as when riding a plane or going on a scuba diving activity. While most of the time, this condition can be manageable, severe pain, tinnitus or ringing in the ears, and vertigo, among others, can be present. Be sure to see your doctor should the symptoms persist.

To prevent this from occurring, whenever you are in flight, be sure to yawn occasionally or take deep swallows. Earplugs are also helpful. You can even chew gum and drink water. Never sleep when the plane is either taking off or landing. As you sleep, pressure builds up in your ears.

Remedies

1. *Valsalva Maneuver*

    This method is useful in letting air out your ear. To do this, press your nose with mouth closed and blow it (while still covering your nose).

2. *Warm Compress*

   Press your affected ear against a warm towel to open your blocked ear.

#8 Clogged Ears

Have you experienced hearing less like you are becoming a bit deaf or hearing windy sounds? Is it as if some liquid or mucus is present? For some, it could be a real hearing disability, but, in most cases, it could be because of a clogged ear. Your ears become clogged when the ear canal becomes blocked as when you have colds, and it is not just annoying but painful too.

Remedies

1. *Steam Inhalation*

   If you have colds, one way to get rid of your clogged ears is by inhaling the steam. As steam gets through your nostrils, mucus, including ear wax, is loosened up, thereby relieving the ears. Bring to boil a pot of water. Remove the pan from the stove once steam starts to come out. Place a towel on your head to secure the steam. Inhale as you bow your head towards the steam. Be sure to lock your hair, especially if it's long so that it would not touch the water.

2. *Take a Hot Shower*

   Hot showers for about 10 minutes can effectively relieve clogged ears too.

3. To eliminate bacterial infection that caused the clogging of your ears, you can mix equal amounts of apple cider and alcohol. Using a medicine dropper, you can have a few drops on your ear as you lie on one side. Allow it to sit for 10 minutes and use a cotton bud to remove whatever dirt or ear wax. Do the same with the other ear if it is clogged too.

4. *Valsalva Maneuver*

   Same with having an airplane ear, you can also use this to unclog your ear. It would help if you remembered that you would potentially damage your eardrum when doing this will not blow too hard.

5. *Olive Oil Lubricant*

Ear wax must have hardened and caused the clogging of your ear. Lubricate and soften it with olive oil for easy removal. Note that you should use pure olive oil. Warm it a little and with the use of a dropper, have a few drops on the affected ear while you lay on the side. Never raise your head. Leave it for 10 minutes and clean your ears slowly with a cotton bud.

#9 Dry Mouth

Dryness in most parts of the body, especially in the mouth area, can be caused mostly by medications and drugs used to treat asthma, diarrhea, acne, hypertension, obesity, and a lot more. Lack of saliva characterizes this condition, which is medically known as xerostomia. Smoking can also cause dryness.

Remedies

1. *Aloe Vera*

Aloe Vera is also helpful in treating dry mouth issues. Juice up and drink Aloe Vera juice daily. Use this as a mouthwash. Aside from that, Aloe Vera gel is likewise beneficial to lubricate the area around your mouth. To apply, use a cotton swab and leave it there for 10 minutes before rinsing it off with cold water. This should be done thrice daily.

2. *Lemon and Honey*

Lemon has a lot of benefits. It can cure bad breath problems, increase appetite, and stimulate the production of saliva. Mix a few drops of honey and half a lemon to a glass of water. Make this your drink for the entire day. Drinking pure lemonade is recommended, too, along with using lemon as a mouth rub. If you decide on this last option, sprinkle some salt on a slice of lemon and rub it on your tongue. This will help enhance your taste buds.

3. *Grapeseed Oil*

Grapeseed Oil is rich in vitamin E and moisturizing properties that are necessary to heal dry mouth issues. Vitamin E can effectively cure mouth sores. Rub grapeseed oil inside your mouth, including your tongue, with the use of your fingers. Let it stay overnight and rinse the following morning. Do this daily during bedtime.

4. *Ginger Tea and Honey*

Ginger is effective in retaining fresh breath and stimulating saliva production. Consume 2 cups daily for better results. You can also cut a small piece of ginger and chew it slowly.

#10 Sore Throat

Sore throat is characterized by irritation, pain, or itchiness in the throat. You can also notice hoarseness in your voice, which can last for more than a week. Since it is painful, you find it hard to take in food and drinks, which gets even worse when you force it. This is also accompanied by patches on the tonsils and swollen neck glands. In some instances, you can suffer from fever when having a sore throat.

Allergies, bacterial or fungal infection, a sudden change in weather/environment, and pollution are among the many factors that may cause a sore throat. In severe cases where swollen tonsils block the throat, call the doctor right away.

Remedies

1. *Salt and Warm Water Gargle*

   Preparing warm water and salt gargle is perhaps the oldest treatment for sore throat. This does not only soothe your aching throat but also helps kill bacteria and breaking down secretions.

2. *Peppermint Spray*

   Peppermint oil can help relieve a sore throat as it contains menthol, which effectively calms coughs, including sores in your throat. Aside from that, it thins out thick mucus allowing easy passage. Studies have backed up its antibacterial, antiviral, and anti-inflammatory properties.

   To prepare your very own peppermint spray, mix a drop of peppermint oil to two tablespoons of raw honey, two tablespoons of peppermint tea, and a tablespoon of warm water. Transfer the mixture to a spray bottle and start spraying it into your mouth, focusing on the throat. Refrigerate the remaining spray to last for months.

3. *Honey and Tea*

    Honey and tea work well as a sore throat cure. Honey is a fast-wound healer. This combination is also good for coughs. Take 2-3 cups daily.

4. *Echinacea and Sage Spray*

    These are effective sore throat relievers too.

5. *Sage Tea*

    Sage tea contains antiseptic and antibacterial properties also. Gargling or drinking can cure any oral inflammation, including coughs and sore throat.

Chapter 3

Frowned Upon Skin Issues

The skin is what covers our entire body from head to toe. It is also very delicate. It shows how healthy you are, by the way, it glows. It can also define your age. Looks can be deceiving at times, and having healthy, glowing skin can give you a few steps backward than your actual age. So, it is but essential to be mindful of it, give it some pampering like the rest of your body. Here is a list of some of the most frowned upon skin issues and their remedies.

#1 Boils

Skin abscess or boil is a common skin infection and is contagious. They appear as bigger versions of ordinary pimples but are firmer, harder, and contain pus in the middle. It looks like an eye. This pus is a collection of white blood cells formed to fight off infection. It becomes increasingly tender over time and is painful. Boils appear in any part of the body –

arms, breast area, head or scalp, face, buttocks, thigh, back, underarms, and groin.

Remedies

1. *Salted Warm Water Compress*

   Adding salt to warm water will speed up the healing process and decrease the pain around the area. To do this, prepare a basin with warm water and add a tablespoon of salt. Soak a washcloth on the bowl, squeeze the water out and press it on the affected area for 15 minutes. Repeat this procedure thrice daily.

2. *Garlic Spot Treatment*

   Create a paste out of 2 crushed garlic cloves and a few drops of water. Apply it directly on the affected area and wrap it with a clean cloth. Make sure that you do not put too much garlic (just enough) else you will burn your skin. Leave it for 15 minutes and repeat this thrice daily. Consumption of garlic is likewise encouraged as this spice contains high anti-viral, anti-inflammatory, and anti-bacterial properties, all of which are needed to heal boils faster.

3. *Tea Tree Oils*

Tea tree oil is a known remedy for ringworms and psoriasis due to its antibiotic, antifungal, and antimicrobial properties. With that, it has also been found to be effective in treating boils. Before applying, make sure you have washed the affected with warm water. If you use undiluted tea tree oil, be sure to observe whether you have developed irritation. If so, stop using it in full strength and dilute it in water. Secure it with a bandage and repeat this process thrice daily for faster healing.

4. *Onion Mask*

Onion contains flavonoids and potassium salts, all of which having anti-inflammatory properties. Onions are known to have a long-standing medicinal proof for various conditions. They are good antioxidants too. As it has disinfectant and anti-inflammatory properties, it is, therefore, useful in treating boils. To use this remedy, apply onion slices on your boils and keep them in place with a bandage. Leave it there overnight for faster healing.

5. *Onion Wash*

If you plan to have onion as your wash, you can do so by boiling onions in a pot of water. Take them out once the amount of water has reduced to half. Remove the onions with a strainer and allow the water to cool. This can now be used to wash your boils.

#2 Hickeys

Love bites or kiss marks as it is called; this results from excessive sucking or aggressive biting, especially on soft parts of the skin, causing the capillaries to break and bleed. These can appear on the neck, chest, or arms—that why they look red or purplish patches. Although you can conceal them with make-up, they can be quite embarrassing as healing take longer.

Remedies

1. *Aloe Vera*

Containing anti-inflammatory and soothing properties, Aloe Vera hastens the healing of ruptured capillaries. Take an Aloe Vera leaf, then scrape its gel out. Place the gel directly on the hickeys. The application should be three times a day for faster healing.

2. *Consumption of Vitamin K-Rich Foods*

Broccoli, brown rice, fish oil, spinach, and soybeans are rich in vitamin K, which you need to ingest when having hickeys. Take in vitamin K-rich foods to prevent blood clotting or coagulation. The healing process hastens as it reabsorbs pooled blood.

3. *Cold Compress*

Same when bruised, it is advisable to always use a cold compress to stop the bleeding and constrict ruptured capillaries. Blood clots break and are separated apart. Press it on the hickeys for 15 minutes, and if you do not have a cold pack, you can wrap ice cubes in a paper towel. Avoid pressing the ice directly on your skin to avoid getting an ice burn.

Remember those metal spoons for your eye bags? You can also use them here. Wrap chilled metal spoon with a thin cloth, then rub it lightly on your kiss mark at least thrice daily.

4. *Banana Peel*

   Banana peels can also help in removing hickeys. Be sure to cut them into sizes that are similar to the hickeys, as this would serve as a spot treatment and leave it there for half an hour. Do this at least three times daily until hickeys are gone.

5. *Peppermint Oil*

   As peppermint improves blood circulation, this is good for hickeys. Gently apply to the area once or twice daily but do not overdo to avoid irritation.

Conclusion

You have finally reached the last part, and for that, I want to thank you again for purchasing this book!

Every single day, you face different situations that mostly involve your body. It could be as simple as these common health problems that may seem tolerable and without potentially harming yourself, or it can be as complicated as having a deadly disease like cancer. For most of us, we overlook whatever we have until such time when someone would notice it or if the condition worsens or gets complicated. Even a simple fungal infection must be treated right away to prevent it from being severe or spreading to other body parts.

Health is wealth. Do not just hide those imperfections like acne or puffy eyes. Concealers and makeups are not the answer; better aim for remedies that can address your health problems.

Like many people, I know you would want to look young, fresh, and flawless. This book contains various do-it-yourself home remedies that can surely help you deal with common health issues. Go ahead and start examining your skin and body. Look at every inch and begin trying these natural remedies at the comforts of your home. They are made from natural ingredients, so you can be sure that they are safe and easy to use.

I hope you enjoyed reading this book and be able to share this with others who need it too.

www.ingramcontent.com/pod-product-compliance
Lightning Source LLC
Chambersburg PA
CBHW062017280526
45787CB00005B/2143